AF773672

Good Health

Tips for a Better Living

Compiled and developed by
G.C. Jain

Rupa . Co

Rupa & Co
7/16 Ansari Road, Daryaganj
New Delhi 110 002

Copyright © Rupa & Co 2000

An Original Rupa Paperback
First published 2000

Compiled and developed by G.C. Jain

Cover design: Arrt Creations

Typeset by
Nikita Overseas Pvt Ltd
19A Ansari Road
New Delhi 110 002

Printed in India by
Gopsons Paper Ltd
A-14 Sector 60
Noida 201 301

ISBN 81-7167-417-8

Introduction

The Good Health Guide has been designed to help the reader combat minor everyday health problems. The book is not meant to be a replacement for your physician. The home-made remedies herein will, however, enable you to deal with an emergency before you are able to get medical aid. Do not take any warning signs lightly. They may be an indicator of a worsening condition. We sincerely hope that this guide succeeds in providing some relief to the user.

As one grows older, the zinc, copper, iron, calcium and chromium content in the body goes down. These can be replaced by multivitamin tablets.

Aging results in insomnia, mental confusion and various kinds of anaemia. Doses of vitamin B1, B6 and B12 have been known to be effective.

Rinse your mouth seven to eight times after every meal and massage your gums with the middle finger of your right hand. It will help clean and wash small food particles from the grooves between your teeth.

Place a small onion on your aching tooth. It may relieve you of your pain.

Do not scrape carrots before eating them. Washing them thoroughly is good enough.

Always opt for soft tooth brushes. Hard brushes may scratch your gums, inviting infections.

Inculcate good eating habits in children. Three meals a day are enough for a child. Encourage him to chew the food he eats, and advise him to eat slowly.

Old people do not pass enough urine. They should avoid high protein diets and sodium (salt) as it puts extra strain on the excretory functions of the kidneys.

During hot, humid and sultry weather, socks should be changed atleast twice a day. Nylon socks aggravate foot infection. If you sweat more in that area, switch to cotton socks.

Women should dry their feet and the area between the toes. They should not walk around with wet feet in the house and allow fungus to develop between the toes.

Remember to fill your mouth with water whenever you wash your face or splash the eyes. It will keep your eyes healthy.

Add some baking soda to your bath water to sooth itching or minor skin rashes.

Minor dysentery troubles can be relieved by eating a single banana, or rice with curd.

Drinking 8-10 glasses of water everyday will prevent kidney or bladder stones.

Noodles, spaghetti and macaroni may taste good. They, however, lack fibre and their vitamin content is destroyed due to excessive use of salt, sugar and preservatives. Do not consume too often.

Place rugs in your home instead of wall to wall carpets. Carpeting traps dust, pollen and insects, creating a health menace in the house.

Biting insects prefer dark colours. They will bite you less if your bed linen and night clothes are white.

Avoid poisonous bug sprays. Spray boric acid mixed with water in your kitchen. It helps you get rid of cockroaches, ants and termites.

Washing hair with a paste of cooked black gram (urad) and fenugreek (methi) increases the hair growth, prevents graying and cures dandruff.

Relieve yourself as soon as you feel the urge. Do not delay passing of urine, as it strains your body.

Soak your legs in warm water just before going to bed to induce a sound sleep.

Snoring can be controlled by sleeping on the stomach.

Do not pull the covers over your head while sleeping even in winter. One needs more oxygen and, therefore, the nose should not be covered at all.

A firm mattress and hard bed are much better for your back than soft ones.

Calcium is not only good for the bones but also reduces the cholesterol level.

Never use nasal drops for more than 7-10 days to decongesting your nose. Visit your doctor if the problem persists.

Cabbage in its raw form is known to alleviate the discomfort of constipation. Its juice is also a good cure for duodenal ulcers. It has excellent therapeutic and curative benefits. Wash every leaf well before use.

Sitting in the car with your back touching the seat during long journeys is harmful. Instead, touch the back of the seat with the sides of your body. Also, get out and walk a little, halting for a few minutes occasionally.

If you are an arthritis patient, limit your fat intake. Keeping your weight low is of prime importance in such a condition.

Diabetic patients usually take a little extra dose of insulin or anti-diabetic drugs whenever they eat sweets or fried food. This is dangerous and can lead to low blood sugar and create an emergency situation.

A warm tea bag can stop bleeding from small cuts.

If you have dry skin, avoid hot water baths. If cold water does not suit you, apply mustard oil on your body before bathing.

Whenever you feel that you have eaten excessively, take a spoonful of black mustard (rai) with water. It will cure indigestion.

Soak 10 almonds overnight, blanch and grind them into a paste. Mix one teaspoon of milk cream (malai) and one teaspoon of coconut oil. Apply the paste on your face and massage for fifteen minutes before bathing. You will see the glow on your face within a few days.

In case of a mild sore throat, gargle with warm salted water specially before going to sleep.

If you enjoy good health, walk up the staircase. Avoid using lifts and escalators for a floor or two.

Walk as much as you can comfortably but briskly. A walk after dinner is a must.

Eat at least one fruit everyday.

Bananas are a good source of potassium.

Eating guavas can rid you of constipation.

When standing, distribute your body weight on both legs.

Foods with a high fat content have a disastrous effect on your power of concentration. You may find yourself mentally slow and having poor judgement.

Groundnuts contain more protein than meat and eggs.

When dieting, do not try to lose more than five kilos a month. It will not only make you weak but also add to your weight immediately when you resume your normal diet.

Shoes should be chosen so that they cover and protect your feet. Make sure your toes rest comfortably in their natural position. Buy them only in the evenings as that is the time when the feet are heaviest and a little swollen.

Fill a green bottle with water and keep it in the sun for a few days. Wash your eyes with this water to give relief to your eyes.

Put some slices of kheera (cucumber) on the eyelids for some time and your eyes will feel refreshed.

If the cuticle (the skin just below your nails) is dry, cracked or cut, apply some antibiotic cream or vaseline on them before going to bed.

Generally speaking, a dry climate is better suited to an asthmatic person than a humid one. He or she should try to live away from the sea coast.

Children sometimes are administered bitter medicine which they do not like. You can crush the medicine and mix with water or honey for it to taste better.

If you are suffering from peptic ulcer, it is advisable to take refrigerated milk without sugar three or four times a day.

Do not take Aspirin and Ibuprofen with fruit juices, coffee, tea or aerated drinks as this may worsen the condition.

Apply some lemon juice mixed with sugar on your hair. Wash it off after 4-5 hours. It is a good remedy for dandruff.

It is a common habit to discontinue treatment the moment the patient gets relief. Always complete the course of a medicine as per the advice of the doctor.

Bend backwards and stretch your body to the maximum as often as you can. Also turn and twist your body on the right and left side. It will keep your body supple and healthy.

Neem (margosa) is an excellent disinfectant tree. Grow it in your house premises if you can.

For minor itching problems boil some neem leaves and mix it into your bath water, which should be lukewarm.

Applying a small amount of mustard oil or vaseline about half and inch deep in your rectum will save you from piles throughout your life. If you already suffer from piles do this everyday after easing yourself and feel the relief.

For minor burns or skin rashes and irritations apply the gel of Aloe Vera (*ghee-kaur — guar patha*) on it several times.

Ajwain (bishopseed) is good for gas and pains. Half a spoon after meals helps digestion.

Eat lots of sprouts, preferably uncooked.

Washing your hair with soap or shampoo every day will increase the dandruff. Shampoos are more harmful because they contain acid.

Wash dry hair once and oily hair twice a week. Use brushes instead of combs.

Do not squeeze pimples or whiteheads on your face. It aggravates the problem and may lead to infections.

Amla (acerola) is a great source of vitamin C even in its dried form. Take a spoon of the powder with milk or warm water. Vitamin C is a sure anti-aging formula. It also helps in resisting colds, bad colds, bad throat, hay fever and allergies.